The Sun-Room

A Memoir

Jess Watts

¶

Published by Linen Press, London 2025

8 Maltings Lodge, Corney Reach Way, London W4 2TT

www.linen-press.com

© Jess Watts 2025

A CIP catalogue record for this book is available from the British Library.

Cover art: Shutterstock
Cover Design: Jess Watts
Typeset by Zebedee
Printed and bound by Lightning Source
ISBN: 978-1-0683417-0-0

About the Author

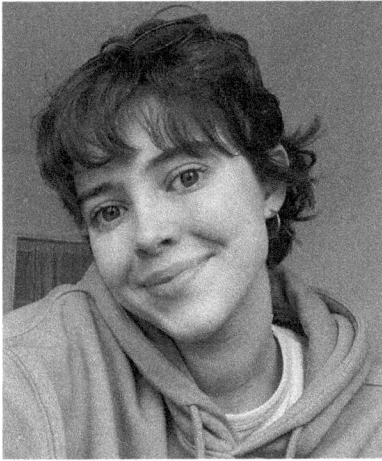

Jess has been writing stories since childhood. Her first completed work, aged eight, was a fully illustrated Horrid Henry fanfiction, lovingly laminated by her grandma. Eighteen years on, *The Sun-Room* – a prose poem memoir about chronic illness grief – is her debut publication.

In 2020, Jess graduated from UEA with a degree in English Literature with Creative Writing. She lives in South London where, health permitting, she writes, reads, and enjoys or despises football.

www.jesswattsauthor.com

Introduction

Editor, Lynn Michell

Jess has written a fabulously original prose poem in which she rages against being felled by an illness that has no agreed name, no treatment, no prognosis. As her life shrinks from university campus to her bedroom, her physical illness is but one part of the story as she tells us how it feels to be robbed, in her buoyant early twenties, of her present and her future. Of possibility. *Sickness has reduced my promised potential to a wasteland.* We need her words – poetic, shocking, strong – to tell the truth about disability.

As someone who lost many years to ME/Chronic Fatigue/Call-it-what-you-will, Jess's writing, twenty-five years down the line from my own full recovery, hits me with its heart-breaking truth. In a few lines, I am back there, in the ME Ghetto, unable to find my way out. The emotional aftermath is not buried after all but follows me into a life rebuilt. To work with Jess has been a surprise and a joy. My editing has, I hope, been as considered as always, and I've loved this collaboration with an exceptionally talented author, but under Jess's prose hangs the underbelly of remembering, and that's still a very dark space.

My long years of being housebound began with my birthday party. What followed was a flu-like virus that affected a good proportion of those who came to my house, many from the same Edinburgh University academic department. Both my sons and I became ill. So did lecturers and post-grads. And the Head of Department. And the administrator. We fell like flies and didn't get up again, but no one in the medical profession was interested in this outbreak. Of necessity, we turned to one another for support and to hang on to our sanity in the face of ignorance and disbelief. Aged six, one of my sons missed every other year at primary school. He was a limp rag, a white-faced outline of the boy he once was, but in a hospital bed, a consultant diagnosed him as dyslexic because he reversed the 'd' above his drawing of a teddy. This consultant went on to become the lauded, leading proponent of CBT and graded exercise, a punishment not a treatment. You don't ask someone halfway through chemotherapy to get up and jog round the block. At my son's school, a PE teacher did ask a boy, similarly ill, to run round the perimeter of the school playing field because ME was just skiving, wasn't it? That boy spent the next year in bed. My son spent four years of his adolescence in bed. I mean *in bed*. At a stretch, he could tolerate watching football on TV, and that left him trembling and soaked in sweat. We watched a lot of football during those years. He was accused of being a school phobic and in my medical notes I saw I'd been given the label Munchausen's syndrome by proxy which means I was keeping my son at home and pretending he was ill because it suited me.

There are many names for this little understood illness – ME, Chronic Fatigue Syndrome, Fibromyalgia and recently Long Covid. Are they all the same? We don't know because there is so very little funding for research. In the 1980s when we all became ill, it was the Cinderella illness and it still is. I had to give up my work as an academic ethnomethodologist (listening to other people's stories), but as I pulled out of the worst, I wrote about an illness whose personal story was largely untold. Then, I easily found thirty people within a ten-mile radius who were ill or very ill, and I recorded interviews with all of them. These were lives reduced to rubble. The result is *Shattered: A Life with ME*, published by HarperCollins.

It's thirty years between *Shattered* and *The Sun-Room*. In 2021, Covid came, and in its wake, Long Covid, a recognised post-viral fatigue state following an infection from Covid-19. Jess was not tested for Covid-19 so she does not know if that triggered her current illness, but the time frame is right. Long Covid symptoms, such as a wired exhaustion unlike normal tiredness, an inability to tolerate sensory input, chronic pain, headaches, and brain fog, may 'closely mimic those seen in ME/CFS'.[1] There is no diagnostic blood test for either illness and so guessing prevalence is more an art than a science,

---

1 https://www.gov.uk/government/statistics/national-flu-and-covid-19-surveillance-reports-2024-to-2025-season/

but one recent UK study estimates that it affects 2 million people[2], while a US study puts it at 18 million.[3] Here is not the place for an exhaustive description of post-viral illnesses, but what does need to be said loud and clear is that in the forty years between my illness and Jess's, there are still only hypotheses about the causes and as yet there is no treatment.

Jess's account of how this illness can halt a life needs to be published. I know of no other personal story that reaches to the bare bones of the all-pervasive suffering that comes when a toxic virus takes up permanent residence in what was a healthy body. Jess grips the suffering by the throat and, despite her own weakness, her own limitations, she rages at what she has lost. She writes with a raw, bleak and beautiful energy as she rails at the unfairness of it and the lack of an ending for herself, and for all others who wait to see if their lives can be reclaimed from the wreckage. Her bravest sentences are her last as she puts aside her anger and sits in a small, sun-lit space.

---

2 national-flu-and-covid-19-surveillance-report-17-october-week-42

3 https://www.theguardian.com/world/2024/mar/15/long-covid-symptoms-cdc

For

Ciara, Julie & Kirsty

Thank you for waiting for me

Note

For years, the Ernest Hemingway quote, 'Write hard and clear about what hurts', was stuck to the wall above my desk, long before I understood the liberty in that instruction.

The following story comes from journal entries and iPad notes, written over two years from spring to spring after I was diagnosed with chronic fatigue syndrome.

The increasing permanence of this illness utterly devastated me – and it still does. Sorrow is not confined to the past tense, but I promise that these pages have not been abandoned to despair. My hope is that, in reading, you witness both pain and transformation, sometimes simultaneous, sometimes one as a consequence of the other.

I have written hard and clear about what hurts and, in the process, what hurts has re-written me.

I have written, without intention, a love letter to the destructive, *miraculous* potency of words.

'But once the vessel cracks, the light can get in. The light can get out.'

Paper Towns, John Green

1.

Grieving for yourself is a
kaleidoscope
of invisible colour.

I am trying out a wheelchair in an air-conditioned shop, surrounded by pictures of smiling, elderly actors, and I don't believe that this is real. I am sitting in an old school room, trying to convince an occupational therapist that I need a disabled badge, while Mum cries beside me, and I don't believe this is real. *This isn't really me*, I want to tell the shop assistant and the therapist, *there has been some terrible mistake. I was healthy and employable, just like you.*

Mum drives me down the same roads I used to walk on. I wind down the windows and reach for a freedom outside of my body – I see myself, headphones on, strolling by and can't decide if I want to protect or kill her. The envy has found its way into my reflection. I scroll through old pictures and hate who I was: my pretty hair and pretty makeup in a selfie before a night out, a video of me singing along to Avril Lavigne with a Strongbow in my hand. I hate her with a depth I didn't know was possible.

We look nothing alike now. My long, thick waves have been replaced by a buzz cut. It thrills me to know that my younger self would be horrified to see what her hair has become because I want the shock to shock us, shock everyone. This is what has happened to me, this is the change I have experienced. I am not the same and I never will be.

I have been broken.

Split, Croatia.

A sleepy, candyfloss sunset lay atop the cruise ships and fishing boats in the harbour. I don't remember the smell but I like to think it was the smell of the sky.

We had spent the day island hopping and stood with all the other sun-drunk tourists, under the palm trees wrapped up in fairy lights.

We piled onto a coach, our disparate cultures spilling and singing into the aisles. Someone, I think it was us, started that song from Shrek and a group of boys from Belgium joined in at the *looking kind of dumb* part.

My face was cracked open in that magic, hysterical, electric happiness that swept up everyone and everything.

When the Spice Girls rang out over the bar speakers, we knew almost every word to the rap, and when a woman appeared with a violin and started playing The Game of Thrones theme, we all cheered, the whole bar, and thrust our drinks towards a ceiling scattered with rainbow lights.

It's a pearlescent memory that my mind glorifies, as an oyster does its treasure. I marvel at it; I marvel at *me*. Like the laughter that burst out of me as we skipped down the street towards the 24-hour bakery, feet aching from dancing for hours and hours. I chose a croissant with buttercream and encouraged my friend to *slap* her beastly mosquito bites, not itch them, between bites of my 3am pastry.

I thought I was the closest I've ever been to the whole world. I tasted it on the watered-down alcohol, more sugar than ethanol, and heard it on the languages that fizzed around me in the club bathroom. There was nothing bigger, nothing more *real* than what I held in my tilting, tipsy gaze.

I was sparkling youth.
I was.
I was.
I was.

The past tense haunts me. I see it on the mouths of my friends as they speak of the present.

You were.
You were.

I hear choral song; the monastic chants of minds and bodies that have slowed and contorted beyond our control.

We were.
We were.

I sing with them. I cry with them.

The sick inhabit a shadow-realm where the healthy don't want to tread. They prefer not to find us, to wait until we've overcome our ailments and stand atop Mount Everest with a smile that declares Look How Strong I Was To Get Through This.

Not everything is an inspiring sound-bite story for the healthy to consume and the sick to aspire to. It's not a battle with a winner; disease doesn't pick an opponent to challenge to a duel.

Do something grand and extraordinary to make your sickness relevant, says society. We want our disabled shiny and productive.

I try not to listen to these voices but sometimes, they sound too much like me.

There is no cure for the kind of exhaustion that sleeps inside your cells. Doing takes energy: walking, talking, listening, eating, watching TV, washing, dressing, and every other action. It is a sickness that requires *being,* but being in a society of doing feels like setting yourself down to die.

My blood work comes back normal, my blood pressure is normal. I must be wearing normal inside out. Some doctors prescribe exercise for ME/CFS sufferers, an instruction that can push fragile bodies until they snap, permanently damaged. Medical professionals are frustrated by the inconclusiveness of this condition, just as we are, and take their minds and money elsewhere.

We can't move on from our bodies. Now, the thing to do is to do nothing: to rest. My mind does not want to rest. It riots against the inertia of sickness. It is alive with grief, guilt that my grief is inadequate compared to the horror on the news, grief that is offset against the privileges I still retain. They ping against the walls of my mind, incessant, popping candy thoughts. I experience all of them, lying here, in this room of heartbreak and sun.

'When I'm healthy again,' I say to a friend, as we plan our fictitious adventures in Seoul, South Korea. We're on the same plane of existence here: a future that neither of us can be sure of, distant enough to glisten in possibility.

I don't know if I believe I will ever be healthy again, or maybe I believe so fiercely because I refuse to believe that I'm not. My existence has to hang somewhere in this balance but I'm a resistance force, my dreams and ambition and anger a barricade of ghosts armed with refusal.

This is not my life. This *can't* be my life. I don't want this life.

Cancelling a flight to America cracked open grief like the spine of a novel, the pages flat across my bed, reality in a double-page spread.

It was holding me up, the false promise that I could do this wild thing and visit my best friend even though I could barely leave my house.

'I probably won't be able to go,' I texted, along with the screenshot confirmation of flight tickets. 'But let's just scream about it!!!!!'

I knew it was a lie, my *body* knew it, it spoke at night, *you are sick, Jess, let yourself be sick,* but if I acquiesced, I would collapse into grief. The fragile home I'd made for my illness, where I'd inhabit silly, futile futures like flights to America, would be exposed as glittering denial.

First, there was a hollow swell of relief –

Then grief crawled in.

I am frightened.

I am frightened because the hooded figure before me is my reflection. All I thought I would be is in this fatigued face.

Two years ago, I handwrote the following paragraph (pretentiously in the third person). I was spending most hours of the day on Reddit, a habit that left me hollowed out.

She takes nothing but her pages. Here, she can be anywhere. Technology has filled her need for rest; she reads the thoughts of others to smother the dull noise of her own. They aren't stories but inflations of her own, spherical existence where everything is mirrored and light bounces between. She is happiest now searching for such slippery things as words. She doesn't need to tame them – she has run with them for years, escaping the mirrors. To rid herself of her reflection is a necessity for fleeing. And she must do what her physical body cannot.

Now, the mirror is all I can see.

2.

I have turned myself inside
out to try to find the words.
Beneath my skin is a scream.

Eight o'clock every weekday evening, second year of university, I'd be stretched out on the saggy leather sofas to watch *The Vampire Diaries*. In the CW masterpiece, when people are turned into vampires, their worst personality traits are magnified.

'What would yours be?' asked my housemate, from where she lay star-fished on the carpet in the dark, listening to Swedish spa music.

I thought about my own personality, how I could pick it apart and offer it up as victim. 'Maybe... jealousy?'

Jealousy is deleting the Instagram app because pixel-perfect square lives exhaust me.

Jealousy is the sharp pinch in my stomach when looking over a classmate's shoulder at their paper and seeing a mark higher than mine.

Jealousy is containable.

Envy is polluting.

Envy is a colour and a scent and a taste.

A heavy, sickly cloying thing, like treacle, that solidifies under your skin and spreads over your rib cage and crawls up your neck until you can't look at the world without choking.

I'm most ashamed of my envy. This vampiric illness has made envy terrifying.

It is not yet 9am and the sun is filling my room. I hear the front door close and understand that it's a beautiful day and that Mum has driven to the seaside with my grandma. The sun taunts me. I want to shut it out. I can't accept the joy of sunlight on my pillow, not when there are people out there experiencing more of it.

When Mum comes back home to the daughter she knows will be there day after day after day, anger will coil and spit within me.

Is this the ugly root of my heart? I envy harder than I love and burn everyone to the ground so that I may have some company in the embers.

I look in the mirror and see a monster who wears grief in talons and fangs. I am hideous, I say out loud, I am hideously crippled by this miasma of longing.

I *bathe* in it. It soaks my skin and if you were to cut me, I'd bleed envy.

Guilt curls up inside me now. I am an egotist, participating in a solipsistic grief of myself for myself. I know that it *could be so much worse* – even within my own life, it has been *so much worse*. There are weeks when I can't even sit up in bed or lift my hands, let alone write – but I am completely transfixed, made maniacal, by the knowledge that it used to be *so much better.*

My little brother knocks on my door and finds me crying on my bed. He's saying goodbye before heading into the city; I can smell his cologne as he folds his arms around me.

I tell him: 'I love when you're home but it also hurts so much.' He asks me why and I say, 'Because you're a living reminder of everything I can't do anymore.' I look at him in this battleground of love and envy. 'I'm sorry.'

He hugs me tighter. 'I'm sorry too.'

August has come already. The year has rolled in on itself and I am somewhere, squished between the months. I haven't seen a single friend since early spring and my phone is turned off, buried under my Crystal Palace beanies, in the third drawer of that IKEA dresser everyone owns.

I know that separating myself from my friends is an act of self-preservation but it feels like another symptom of sickness. I cannot find it in me to ask about their jobs or new apartments, their relationships or summer plans. Those questions would reveal the envy monster I am trying to tame, the one who avoids a reality I was once part of. Their answers would tear my tongue, then slither, acidic, over the cut. I am holding onto a bleeding heart and the helping hand they want to offer only deepens the wound.

I have taken down the frame of Polaroids in my room: instant moments of joy from holidays abroad, drunken snaps before and after a night of dancing, my eyes a sharp red in the flash, way too many starring Domino's Pizza, my fresher's meal of choice.

I don't know how to explain to my friends that their smiling, frozen faces hurt me. I don't know how to explain it to myself. I *miss* them as I miss myself because we are inextricably entwined.

I was the piss-your-pants laughter in a shitty Premier Inn; I was the terrible attempt at an Australian accent on the Northern Line at 2am; I was the spontaneous dance on the golf course overlooking the London skyline. Are they mourning this loss like I am? – because their friend is dead, and there has been no funeral.

I hate the bitterness in the words I write about people I love. They're the collateral damage of my splintered life and envy has collected the pieces.

I want these friendships, and I want their empathy. But I want them to leave their lives by the door, come in and just lie beside me.

Envy is a colour and a scent and a taste and a sound.

Envy is a howl of anger and I hate that I hurl my scream at these people I love because ME is faceless.

The internet tells me that anger is a secondary emotion. This makes sense to me – I know that my anger is a messy concoction of sadness, hopelessness and fear. I am not typically an angry person. The grief of chronic illness is unearthing pieces of myself I didn't know were there.

But anger makes me feel alive. I have renewed energy: energy to punch a pillow, to scream, to tear a piece of paper into tiny shreds over and over again. The grief fuelling this pseudo-energy is bottomless. My history and my future are in this storm. Soon there will be nothing left of me.

The pen is mightier than the sword but I need my words to cut like a blade. I need to bleed.

Rage is inescapable, in every sinew of my flesh. I can't tear my skin from its bone or rip the beating heart out of my ribcage and sob in the sweet relief of peace because death would take too much. I am so angry; I hold my arm between my teeth and *scream*. I want to release a battle cry but I'm surrounded by neighbours, people everywhere. I slam on the keys of my laptop, the rapid motion already triggering the dormant ache in all my limbs.

I don't know how to do this.

My self-harm was walking beyond my twenty-metre limit. Now, the pain in my legs, my hands, is growing. It's the evil payback for trying to unleash the rage that might one day swallow me whole. I am so angry; I close my eyes and pretend I am a hungry lion sprinting down the African plains in pursuit of a dazzle of zebras. I am a maniacal, deranged super villain swinging her way through a city with a sledge hammer.

I need to be someone else. Anything else.

A colour, a sound, a feeling.

Red hot. Flash. The October sun. I pick up the roll of wrapping paper. I whack it against the leg of my desk over and over and over. My scream vibrates in my throat. My bundled-up dressing gown catches the pain because my neighbours are back from their holiday and I don't want them to hear.

'I'm so angry. I feel so fucking angry again!'

'Well, I can't do anything now! I'm about to go out!' And Mum slams the front door and flees to my cousin's eighth birthday celebration.

I've only managed to see my cousin once since she turned seven.

A Google search: 'Help with Intense Anger'

The following paragraph is from Mind:

Do something to distract yourself mentally or physically – anything that completely changes your situation, thoughts or patterns can help stop your anger escalating. For example, you could try: putting on upbeat music and dancing, doing something with your hands, like fixing something or making something.

What the fuck are you supposed to do when you can't change your situation because you carry it with you? My rage is trapped within my body and my body is the cause of my rage. I can only wait to bleed out, waiting, always waiting, for the red to dull to blue.

This is when I cry.

3.

I am unravelling in losses like
ribbons
piled up around my feet.

Curled up on the bed, like a half-formed full stop, I am crippled by a single desire.

I want to wear a graduation gown. I want the stupid hat and cape and smile, all pretty in a dress and wedge heels. I want to wear the old version of myself, except that she's not old, she's shiny and hopeful.

It's her graduation.

They'll call her name and she'll walk across the stage and shake a hand sticky with the sweat of her fellow graduates. Someone whoops and it's her Mum and her best friend, maybe even the boyfriend she thought she wanted at twenty-one in that strange summer of twenty-twenty. She is radiant, her degree is radiant; the future, that fucking radiant oyster of a future, is hers for the taking.

But this is real:

Dad has driven back early from my little brother's graduation to keep me company. He shows me pictures of a twenty-one-year-old in a stupid hat and cape and a face split open in a grin. At first, I am grinning too because I love my brother and I love his happiness, but then, as the pictures keep coming and I see all the other students in their stupid hats and capes and dresses and suits and shoes with wedge heels and families and girlfriends and boyfriends and achievements and future, I excuse myself to the bathroom, sit down on the floor and cry.

I am an unfinished sentence.

GCSE Results Day. A-Level Results Day. A paper Degree certificate in the post.

It's embarrassing really, how these grades I wore as medals have turned to vapour. The golden destination, the undeniable Success of the dream career is just that: a daydream.

The government wants to know if I am earning enough yet to start paying back my student loan. I tick the box that says Unemployed, and feel like a failure.

I believe in an intangible soul that takes temporary shelter in the body. Even when my limbs are pinned to the bed by fatigue, who I am can still float up, up, up like a balloon. I like this separation – my innate humanness from human skin and bones – because sometimes it dulls the envy.

I have always been fearful of the body. Biology was my least favourite science at school. Staring at a PowerPoint presentation about The Heart would make mine launch against my chest in a frenzy, like it didn't want to know it was made of ventricles and veins and looked like a slimy, bloody lump. It didn't want to know what it really was.

For the first twenty-two years of my life, I had the privilege of a body that rarely malfunctioned. It self-repaired when I had a virus or cold. When I was gripped by physical anxiety, I could whisper this will pass, this will pass until, finally, it did.

Now, within the walls of this body, I am walking on eggshells. A new sound of pain, in my ears, my head, my eyes, my limbs, shatters terror into a million pieces of broken glass beneath my skin.

In pain, there is no air to give my soul flight.

If physical pain could write, those words would be the most visceral lashes against the page – lucid enough for the reader's body to hurt too.

But physical pain can't write because physical pain is annihilating: you shrink to a pressure point or swell to a feverish, frightened heartbeat. There are no words in the grip of pain. There may be words afterwards, but they are substitutes for a thing that can't be translated. These migraines and vertigo spells and body aches and panic attacks are wordless voices. There's no listening, no speaking, no communicating with physical pain, only *being* in it. A verb that has to be experienced to be read as true.

I am grateful for every moment I have words, in my mind or out of it, because that means that pain is a noun again.

The words Crash and Flare are ubiquitous in the lexicon of Chronic Illness. The nebulousness of an invisible sickness is echoed in the nebulousness of this language. Flare is acceptable because when symptoms flare, there is inflammation throughout the body, like a flare of the sun. But the semantics of Crash are not. No poet describes heartbreak as a crash.

Crash denotes a collision: energy that builds and builds at speed then explodes in matter. *Stars* are formed out of collisions. A chronic illness crash is a star-less collapse. Energy runs out long before anything as exciting or creative or material as a collision.

There is no word for the noiseless devastation of texting a friend, a month in advance, that you won't be able to make her birthday again this year. There is no word for the silence of lying in a dark room, the silence of putting down the life you were building, of emptying your hands of hope.

Crash. Transitive verb [Merriam Webster Dictionary]

1. to break violently or noisily
2. to damage in landing
3. to cause a loud noise

One of the places I know best in the world is a stretch of promenade in Penzance in Cornwall. In high tide, waves crash against the sea wall and throw themselves over, spitting seaweed across the pavement and car windows. When we were young, my brother and I would hang onto the railing, watching as the sea swelled, belly full with its next attack. Then, just before the collision, we would run away squealing, hair damp from the spray that chased after us.

The last time I was there, my little cousins stood directly in the splash zone, trembling with cold and anticipation. They ran along the promenade looking for where the biggest crashes would come, when two waves from opposite directions would converge at the steps by the saltwater bathing pool. There, the spray towered higher than the houses across the street and rained down over the heads of passers-by. It was always hilarious to see naive tourists gaping in shock as the sea poured off their clothes.

But for my cousins, each crash of the wave that soaked through their raincoats to their skin was a deliberate invitation to pure *joy*.

There is another definition I find, further down the page:

Crash.
A falling short of one's goals.
Example sentence: *Refused to be discouraged by the crash of her hairdressing business.*

How do I refuse to be discouraged by the crash of a life?

It is cruel when what you love becomes a weapon turned against you. I can't sit at a desk and type stories on my laptop without the words swimming. I am lying on the sofa now, typing on my iPad keyboard through squinted eyes, ferociously pushing the sentences out before the dizziness takes over and my head throbs with the words I want to say.

I ration these words of grief, setting timers to lessen the physical consequences. There are long, imprisoned months when I am unable to write anything, and words spark and dissolve in a firework display only my mind can see – and mourn.

'What do you want to be when you grow up?' was always the easiest question for me to answer. My face brightened with a quiet pride and confidence as I replied to teachers or my parents' friends, who bent their questions toward me from their lofty grown-up heights, 'An author.'

I said it with the same certainty as the boys in my class declared they would be footballers. Except I never outgrew this dream.

My university advisor asked me, aged twenty, the same question, phrased instead as 'After university.' I told him I was writing a book.

'A book?' He looked bemused. 'It's not autobiographical, is it?'

'No,' I replied, defensive, 'it's fiction.'

I ranted to my housemate about the ridiculousness of his question. What could a twenty-year-old English

Literature student possibly have to write about for an autobiography? I assumed he was mocking me, having heard every naive student on the Creative Writing programme tell him *I am writing a book*, and I never went back.

And yet, the first book I have completed is a short memoir on chronic illness grief. It is, Mr Advisor, autobiographical indeed.

Irony, the cheeky bitch.

A writer, unable to write. My identity is a war of clauses.

Some typography on Pinterest makes me stop scrolling: *Don't waste your twenties* in green bubble font on a bright pink background. It repulses me, so I click on it. Immediately, there are more graphics in lurid colours, instructing me to squeeze every drop of *laughter and love and mistake* from this decade.

Your twenties are for trying things out and fucking up this time scribbled on a handwritten note, like a secret passed between us. It's nihilistic – as if *fucking up* has no real consequence – but I want that freedom anyway.

Who decided that being in your twenties should be a pursuit of hedonism, rich in the decadence of unlimited potential and do-overs? No, this is not *being* in your twenties, this is *doing* in your twenties. There is a distinct social, capitalist difference.

Maybe it's because just last century, your twenties were a death sentence, and young, opulent blood was spilled all over Europe and beyond. It soaks the poppy-fields visited by history undergraduates on research trips.

I return to scrolling, feeding my sadness and isolation, until I see something that makes me, finally, close the app.

Your twenties are for falling in love.

Romantic love was always an abstract dream, iridescent with possibility.

Sickness has confined Love to a coffin.

A couple of summers ago, I downloaded a dating app. Not with any true intention to go on a date, I barely saw friends anymore, let alone strangers, but just to see what was out there, to tempt the possibility. Yet with every conversation, I saw the limits of my health laid bare. I was invited to a karaoke bar, a night-time art exhibition at the Tate Modern, and the coffin creaked open and Love floated up like a malevolent ghost with a cruel, twisted mouth. Too sick, was my reply to every message, too sick, too sick, too sick. I deleted the app after a day.

My queerness that has since, cautiously, revealed itself from behind a locked door, is trapped behind another one.

I want to believe that there is someone out there who will lie beside me on my bed, listening to the hum of the radio as the tragedy of illness softens between us.

Mum promises me that there will be; sometimes you have to hide inside someone else's hope and let it carry you.

I feel guilty when Mum absorbs my sadness. Countless times over the last years when I'd been sobbing in anger, she would throw me a jacket and order me to sit with her in the car. If I felt well enough, we blasted our favourite BTS songs and drove around the neighbourhood, pretending to perform, with flailing arms, the lightning-quick rap verses. One spring day, when I was unbearably sad, she drove me to the hill overlooking the racecourse and held me in her arms as I literally screamed. When I'd calmed down, she went to buy me a Mr Whippy ice cream with a 99 flake. I took a selfie of me with the cone, looking miserable, eyes squeezed by tears, with Mum grinning beside me. We laughed at it.

I don't stay stuck in the fissure of heartbreak.

But when she sits on my bed and listens and nods as I tell her everything hurts and nothing feels normal, that I miss my old life and hate everyone who doesn't have to miss it, I want to apologise. I cry to her that I am a small child dependent on her mother. I cry to her that I am an old woman with creaking bones who looks back at youth with a confused longing.

She cooks all my meals; she leaves my breakfast in the fridge before she goes to work each morning.

'Am I a burden?' I ask her, though I know she will reply, 'Don't be silly, I love you,' like she does every time. My chronic fatigue fatigues her heart.

As a child, I was enchanted by Disney's Alice in Wonderland. As an adult, I want to shrink to a size small enough to float away on a lazy-river of these tears, through the keyhole and out to paradise, out beyond my body.

One afternoon, a word came unannounced and forbidden and convulsed against my spirit with the power to break it. But my need brought the word. I *wanted* to break, completely, to be nothing.

'I am a husk,' I whispered.

Hollow, shell, useless, dried up, worthless: a body without meaning.

And then it was out in the air of my room, so ugly, so untrue, that Mum said, quietly, 'I never want to hear you say that again.'

Last night, I dreamed that I ran to meet my childhood best friend in the road between our houses where she used to live and I still do. We hugged so tightly for all the months we'd spent apart, and she told me that she was getting married and I sat on the wall, knocked down by all the life I'd missed during the months I'd been lying on my bed.

Every email begins:

I began to develop chronic fatigue symptoms in 2021. Since then, I have become mostly housebound with this condition, also known as ME, and am unable to work.

I lead with it, like a firm handshake in a job interview. Like it's the most interesting thing about me.

Last year, my celebrity crush intensified into obsession. I ensnared him in the capacious potential of a daydream, me playing God, constructing a perfect life free of illness and limitation. I lived in this daydream for *hours*, exiting only to eat or go to the toilet or scroll on my phone.

We were married. We had a house in Hampstead, my favourite part of London, and a five-year-old daughter who was just about to start school. I saw everything in assiduous detail. The birch tree in the front garden, and the Wendy house painted pastel blue in the back. My daughter had a princess bed with a slide – the very bed I desired as a child – and a sweet, rabbit-shaped bookcase full of picture books my husband and I took turns to read with her. The kitchen was large and light-filled, and French windows stretched across the back wall. Because it was August, we kept them open to the garden decking outside and had BBQs with friends in the sun-soaked evenings.

The following definition is from Harvard Health:

Maladaptive daydreaming occurs when a person engages in prolonged bouts of daydreaming, often for hours at a time, to cope with a problem. The daydreams are often vivid and complex plots that elicit a great deal of emotion. A person becomes so consumed by their daydream they may fail to complete work and other daily tasks, or start to withdraw from friends and family.

I had no work. I had no tasks.

I had my bed. I had my mind.

I did not want to look grief in the eyes – my eyes – and shatter the one coping mechanism that was keeping me together. But every time I left the Hampstead house, and the family I'd designed, the disconnect between that fantasy and my real, empty bedroom was agonising.

This is not helping you. You cannot grieve like this – and if you cannot grieve, you cannot heal.

Resisting the lure of that painless place took immense discipline.

Another life to mourn.

Grief is not quantifiable but I keep trying anyway. I want to figure it out – to reinvent my losses into a mathematical formula which offers a solution or restoration. X amount of loss equals Y amount of grief.

*Person A is able to walk **inside** the house but has become unable to go **outside** without the assistance of a wheelchair. What is Y, the sum of their grief?*

Person B has become unable to walk at all. How much greater is Y for Person B than for Person A?

It strikes me as morbidly hilarious, how my affliction of comparison has spread to here, to grief, when the whole world is soaked with it: big, small, visible, invisible, manageable to paralysing.

History is just loss packaged up.

I am waiting for the other shoe to drop.

It's like wearing black tights at school when a tiny tear becomes a gaping hole by the end of the day and swallows my brother, my parents, and the remainder of my health. I am waiting for the real grief, the grief of a death. I am afraid it will obliterate me.

I think I've set off a domino tragedy when really, my tragedy is so personal, so self-absorbed. I've kissed myself in the mirror and smudged the blood across our twin faces.

Who will bleed next? says Anxiety, from where it lounges in an armchair. *Bad things won't just end here.* It tugs at the fraying fabric of the chair, a years-old habit. *Life is one big shit house.*

My own wound has stretched into the gaping wound of the world. I hear murder and rape and fire on the radio; the life outside my home has grown ugly in terror; my heart pounds in fear as I sit against the bed.

I did not think, when I was living out there inhaling life with full lungs, that these awful things could ever happen to me – just as I did not think I would ever be sick. But the disgustedly privileged seams I've lived in have torn. Fear crawls inside. When Mum leaves the house, I have a quiet certainty that she will die beyond the front door.

Because why shouldn't hideous things happen to me? My immunity has cracked and real life, in its swelling, malevolent colour, oozes around me.

I hold a tiny corner of suffering beneath my fingers. I hold the corner of my duvet.

Without urgency, May has yawned into June. My life is the passing of time. I can't decide if summer nullifies or exacerbates my grief. The warmer air and vitamin D feels good on my skin but in summer, people embrace the world in a new way. In those stretching hours of daylight, a freedom opens up. I think of picnics and BBQs and how London is, at this very moment, alive with tourists, like bees invigorated by beautiful, unfamiliar flowers.

There is a bee in the garden with me here. It buzzes over me to rest on the purple buddleia.

On this day, before the next season in the cycle of seasons unfurls before me, I want to be content. I want to sit in my garden in the company of this little bee.

There is so much peace here: in the rustling of the leaves and my hands on my outstretched legs. I am writing in a notebook – the very act of writing a rare blessing – and my sunglasses have turned everything to a sun-drenched orange.

The millions who currently live in a war zone, maybe grieving the horrific loss of a child, a loss so unbearable that they no longer remember how to hold up their bodies, would embrace this peace like the most treasured friend. I think about this with a confusion of guilt because joy isn't the emotion I want to see when placed against the sorrow of others. I am deeply sad. I am experiencing a tragedy, a quiet one compared to that of humanity, but deafening to me. My losses cannot be soothed by the broken hands of the world.

But when I look up from writing, at the bee, at this peace, I tentatively begin to make a home.

Sitting outside in my garden, on this June day, I am a balance of grief and gratitude.

4.

If this is all I can be, if this is the
only place I can go, there is still
life.

Healing in the mind, as I understand it, is two things:

First, it is not linear. Like stitching up a wound, the needle must go in, out, in, out, over and over again, in a dance.

Second, to heal you must let go.

Like social media, alcohol, skinny jeans, binge watching Netflix, reading physical books (audiobooks are an effective replacement). And intangible things like friendships and plans.

Expectation cannot be relinquished so easily. Expectation is a skin that forms in primary and secondary school, and hardens in university classrooms. Expectation is its own DNA. Separating the self from Expectation is, surely, a genetic impossibility.

Deleting photos is my new hobby. I have thousands and thousands stacked up on my camera roll and I tap the bin icon, again and again, like I'm playing an arcade game. It's surprisingly easy to do. Photos are not living things; they are the carcasses of a moment.

I used to be obsessed with recording moments. For six years, I wrote a few sentences every single day to document where I'd been, who I'd seen, what I'd done. My dedication astounds me now. It was as though I knew that, creeping closer with each year, my ability to chronicle what I did with the people I loved would disappear. So, I held every memory in the eye of a phone lens and in ink. I *gripped* them. Holding is a gentle action; gripping is a fearful one.

I could not bear to lose anything. I collected all these beautiful carcasses and decorated my mind with them.

I like the concept of a moment.

I like the way I can extract it from the word *momentary*: I like the quickness, the impermanence of experience, like a sharp burst of noise.

And yet, it is also a long and languid thing, like silence, like peace.

I like that life can fit inside a single moment, and that life itself is a sequence of moments plural.

I like our human desire to preserve the good moments, and that technology's attempt to immortalise them is an artifice in which we all pretend to believe.

There is, in every moment, a beginning and an end, an opportunity and a death.

Moments are as delicate as butterflies. Sometimes we let them go, sometimes we allow them to rest on a finger. Sometimes we kill them with a pin and admire their past tense beauty.

I like that there are infinite, uncontainable metaphors to describe a moment and that, in finishing this sentence, I have left one and entered another.

The first time I searched #MECFS on Instagram I cried because immediately, hundreds of posts, of *people*, offered me their pain. I recognised the sorrow in their captions as my own; the bed-bound selfies of faces framed by the same migraine strips I wear, almost daily, across my own forehead. There were comments of FUCK CFS in solidarity, an empathy that was as true as a reflection.

I am surrounded by healthy people and I had been holding my broken body against their functioning ones. Finding the sick felt like an exhale. I was witnessing a community who understood, and inhabited alongside me, the minutiae of this loss.

I widened my search to #ChronicIllness, to #Spoonie, to #DisabilityPride and was stunned by the colourful chaos of images singing, screaming, sharing. Disabled advocates with fire in their captions, a rallying war-cry for justice in a system infested with ableism. I found expressions of joy in bright pink, spray-painted wheelchairs with crocheted handle warmers and yellow butterflies around the wheel spokes. It felt like a rebellion against the Instagram I knew, and had grown to loathe, where posts are beautiful renditions of life, even the so-called 'candid' photographs layer to form a pretty artifice. I never stay here long, nor do I post or interact, but I am comforted to know that there is life in those hashtags.

Our sick world is a quiet one, the roar of the healthy drowning us out. The healthy churn the wheel of capitalism and give purpose to government tick boxes.

I was once the same. I did not seek out those other voices, and if I stumbled across them, I would hear them with a detached pity, relieved that it wasn't me. I am ashamed of that. I lived in a bubble-wrapped, naive existence with my belief that if I, or anyone else got sick, we would get better.

I have come to learn that the sick are great architects of the little things. We erect cathedrals from radio broadcasts and audiobooks and from the silence of our daydreams. Skyscrapers reach out of the slow hobbies that are mere pastimes for the healthy but time itself to us. Whole cities exist in the digital constellations that map our collective pain.

In a society of capitalism and hustle culture, where hyper-productivity is your access pass, we have had to unlearn, to let go, and so we construct a new, solitary world in the space left behind.

I am proud to be part of this gentle revolution.

Sadness is the opposite of happiness. Envy is the opposite of contentment. My mind has fabricated an image of dichotomous humans in which we who are dealing with sorrow droop, like parched flowers, in the shadow of the tall, happy and unburdened.

I flick through my journals from 2018 and 2019 and am affronted. Those years shimmer in my memory like a mirage, but what I read, amidst the expressions of joy and abundant living, are paragraphs of intense loneliness, anxiety and rejection. The future was something I feared and longed for; I folded my words around it, I made it the purpose of my present.

Now, my access to that world, both 2018 and the desired future, has become condensed to my sick body. And yet, I still laugh, I still cry at beautiful music, I cheer at football goals and embrace excitement in its smaller, precious doses.

The colours of human emotion bleed together. We are a full, mixed wash in the world's grotty, damaged launderette. We exchange a nod of acknowledgment, amidst the peeling paint walls and the incessant whir of the machines: hurting, hopeful, *human*.

It is spring again, or rather spring is standing on tiptoes, preparing to dive into winter and send it scattering. I am well enough to open my curtains and sit at my window where, outside, the sky is that endless, embracing blue.

The pink blossom tree in the garden is waking up and blue tits, the size of cupcakes, flitter between the branches and snip at the fluffy flower heads. As I watch the petals float to the ground, for a moment, I am distressed.

Then I let it be.

Norwich, England.

If I woke to an open-armed sun on an open-armed day, I would take the bus into the city and spend an hour or two at the cathedral.

I always walked the long route from the bus stop: through the archway and into the courtyard, through the cottage garden with the sprawling wild-flowers, through the gaps between the cars in the cathedral car park, and through the open, iron gate. The instant I crossed the threshold into the cloisters, I was enveloped by a solemn serenity. I slowed my pace; I was entering history.

The cloisters were nearly always deserted. I sat with my back against the stone, legs stretched out along the wall, to read a chapter of one of the week's designated novels. Once, I looked up from my book to a snowstorm of choir boys in white robes who strode past me and entered the cathedral through the unassuming door to my left. A while later, their singing flooded all four corridors, swooping through the cloister archways, over the square courtyard and up towards heaven like a majestic, holy bird.

This was the door I always used to enter the cathedral; I slipped in like a secret.

I love that it opened in the spine of the cathedral. Not the cavernous main chamber, bathed in the playful pinks and purples and greens that emanated from the enormous stained-glass window, but a tiny alcove.

I stepped into it so that the curved walls made me an altar, and began to read the graffiti etched into the stone. This absolutely *thrilled* me. There were initials in a Shakespearean font with dates as old as 1652, and I traced my thumb over the markings, feeling that History was alive in my blood. When I took Dad here and showed him what I'd found, he couldn't believe it.

I walked along the periphery of the main chamber, dipping into rooms dense with the kind of softness that slowed the mind, made a pulse of the pad of footsteps on the cold, hard stone.

Near the back of the cathedral was a candle tree. I lit a tealight and placed it inside the metal case. I watched as an older woman did the same, and wondered what she prayed for.

It was not God I felt closest to in the cathedral, it was people; I walked in the relic of their revelry.

Each time I left through the main entrance and out into the sun, I felt that a restoration had occurred deep within me.

I try a new thing. I stand inside the resurrected detail of this memory and say, 'I'm so pleased that we came here so often. I'm thankful for it.' I have not divided my life into the sterile binary of before and after sickness. I have not disgraced my past self from my present by pronouncing her dead. She is me, I am her, *we* walked the corridors of Norwich Cathedral.

I try thanking more memories.

Thank you that we went to Croatia and danced into the early hours of morning.

Thank you that we studied hard because we loved to learn.

If I can find a way to appreciate the past tense without gripping it, if I can find a way to break my idolisation of the future, I think I may find *me,* whole, in the middle.

In the spine.

Rest was never difficult until my body asked, then begged, then made me do it every day.

By releasing Expectation, I have encountered a soft, surprising moment of peace, when I am lying on the bed, arms outstretched in surrender, and sunshine warms my closed eyelids.

I will try to hold myself with gentleness. Mind and body. A unified whisper of 'us'.

I let my hands go limp against this body's walls. I do the only thing that was asked of me as a baby when life meant breath, nothing more, nothing less.

I will try to hold myself with gentleness.

Nine years old, staring into my bedroom mirror and speaking with a cheesy American accent, I am a child star on the Disney Channel. The pinnacle of success.

Growing up, my grandparents' house was a place for indulgence, for warmth – but also for cultivating jealousy. The Disney girls on the screen were confident and articulate, flipping their curls to a bolt of canned laughter. I longed for the incessant affirmations given by adults; I longed to be rushed around a Beverly Hills set on a golf buggy; I longed for their stardom.

The insularity of childhood struck me then. Beyond this protected sphere was a world of possibility, a world of people who would see me.

By early adulthood, I had developed a clandestine desire to be seen everywhere, not merely as myself but as *all* the selves I could become: to be seen as possibility.

I plucked stares from the air and pressed them between my thumb and forefinger, privately, under the table at a restaurant or in my lap on the underground. I pushed them into my skin with discreet pride.

I enjoyed the distance in a stranger's fleeting glance, the incompleteness of their assessment. I was not yet the prettiest or the smartest or the most unique but I possessed the *possibility*.

'She is very capable' and 'She has great potential' was the feedback I internalised from primary school parents' evenings and throughout my education.

Potential [Miriam Webster Dictionary]
adjective

1. existing in possibility: capable of development into actuality
2. expressing possibility

What I heard from these adults was 'Keep going, because you are not yet enough.'

When my high school English teacher gave me a mark, I needed that mark to mean more than a fraction. I needed the certainty of potential.

I carried a hazy glow around my person, the spectre of a future self that would shift each time I filled out the previous frame so that possibility always obscured the present. Since childhood, I had stored layer upon layer of compliments like a kind of second skin.

It was so heavy: the unsatisfied reality of *the present.*

The day before I made the dating app profile – the one that lasted not even twelve hours before deletion – I asked my childhood best friend to take some photos of me. It was early summer and she pushed me in my 98-year-old great grandma's wheelchair, which Mum had affectionately named the BFF, or Big Fat Fucker, along the street to the only patch of greenery in our neighbourhood. This was almost a year before I started writing about grief, days I spent deep in online escapades and excessive daydreaming, a pseudo-protection that I later realised was suffocation. The idea of connecting with people in the real world invigorated me.

My friend, who was squinting at her phone, barked with laughter. The chair was visible in the background of the photos, like an ungainly photobomb. I laughed too.

'Delete all of them! I don't think I can crop it out.'

Recovering, she said, 'They're going to have to find out soon enough', and nothing seemed funny anymore.

We sat under the dying sun, amidst the long grass, pretending this was the countryside and not a South London suburb. She asked me what the hardest thing was. I told her it was wasted potential.

In a wheelchair, possibility is compressed to the metal frame around my incapable body. For months, I have not felt well enough to go out in a wheelchair but when I did go, there was little pleasure in being seen by strangers. I left their stares in the air, hoping they would dissolve. Instead, they buzzed around me like flies.

You can do this, I told myself over and over as I

cowered. I said loudly to whoever was pushing me, 'It's so weird to have everyone stare at you,' to shame those who stared, to tell them *this is all new to me too, wheelchairs are not my normal.*

My beanie hat was pulled low over my shaved head and my eyes were hidden behind sunglasses. If twenty-year-old Jess had walked past, she would have glanced at me, not recognised me, then looked away. Even if I had removed my sunglasses and our shared eyes had met, she would not have understood that I was her future. She would have looked away. She would have continued walking.

I understand now that the pity and sadness I saw in the eyes of those strangers were the feelings that I was experiencing within my own heart. I pulled out of them what was coiling and hissing and spitting and *breaking* in me.

The next time I can go out in a wheelchair, I will try and say a new phrase to myself. I don't need to sit with complete assuredness and meet every stare with a smile. I don't need to shrivel in the seat, confronted by my own ableist prejudices. I will amend the mantra *you can do this* which has always contained pressure about the future.

You can be this, however, is freedom.

Some people bend their lives to a relentless pursuit of perfection; I have been bending mine to a relentless pursuit of possibility.

That sounds like a good thing. It sounds like something written in a typewriter font and found on Pinterest. It sounds like something to be printed off and stuck to the wall above my desk.

I believed that sickness had stolen possibility, ridding me of any transformative powers. I didn't believe that transformation could take place within a stationary body, hidden from the eyes of the world, with only the sun behind a window to bear witness. I didn't believe that transformation could have an internal, present purpose, separate from external, future Achievement.

Sickness has reduced my promised potential to a wasteland.

I am rudderless.

But perhaps that is the true landscape of being?

I am sitting cross-legged before the mirror, and I'm about to do something unnatural. I'm not used to addressing my reflection in the mirror. It's always been my audience.

'I see you,' I begin. 'Not who you were, or who you thought you'd be, or needed to be, or who you may become.'

Sunlight empties over the carpet.

'I see you here, as you are.'

At night, something magical happens to the view out of the bedroom window. The distant buildings, illuminated against the blue-grey dark, become a great ship on the ocean.

Suddenly, I have a horizon.

Afterword

I vacillate between the colliding emotions of these four chapters.

Sickness is a painful, breaking experience that is, at this moment, an enduring one. I may get better; I may get sicker. I continue to be confronted by losses, by the envy and anger of this grief, but I am committed to returning to gentleness: returning to the Sun-Room where *I* am and where *now* can be.

'We float with the sticks on the stream; helter-skelter with the dead leaves on the lawn, irresponsible and disinterested and able, perhaps for the first time in years, to look round, to look up – to look, for example, at the sky.'
On Being Ill, Virginia Woolf

Acknowledgements

I could not have dreamed up a better home for *The Sun-Room* than Linen Press. The greatest thanks to Lynn Michell for being an empathetic and compassionate editor. This entire process has been such an enriching (and fun!) collaboration. Thank you also to Rosie Pundick for your thoughtful comments and questions during the edit. To everyone at Linen Press, the hours of work you dedicate to creating books is invaluable.

Thank you to my parents for their suggestions, read-throughs and constant encouragement. Mum: thank you for your speedy proof-reading and patience with me as I became a frantic writing whirlwind trying to get the first draft finished. Dad: your enthusiasm over your favourite passages is all a writer could ever want from a reader. I love you both immeasurably (and Aidey, of course).

To the friends who graciously agreed to read *The Sun-Room* when it was an unpublished PDF, thank you. I know I can't be in all of your lives the way I used to be, but I so treasure your comments.